COMPLETE FIBROMYALGIA DIET COOKBOOK

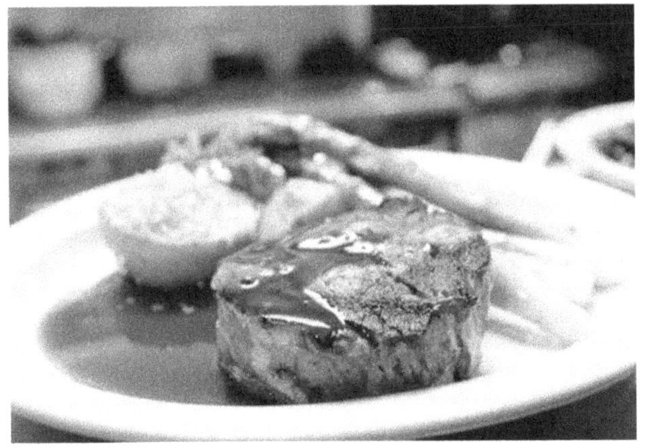

A simple and effective way to manage your symptoms and improve your quality of life to boost your energy and immunity.

KATHLEEN G MARION

TABLE OF CONTENT

INTRODUCTION

Florence, a woman painted in shades of vibrant hues, had become shrouded in a haze of fatigue and pain. Fibromyalgia, an unwelcome guest, had settled in, stealing her energy and dimming her once luminous spirit. Daily tasks felt like monumental climbs, and joy, a forgotten friend. Food, once a source of pleasure, became a minefield of triggers, each bite a potential flare-up.

One day, while browsing a bookstore, a book with an emerald cover caught her eye. "Complete Fibromyalgia Diet Cookbook" whispered hope. Hesitantly, Florence picked it up, the author's words resonating like a forgotten melody. Inside, she discovered a world of vibrant vegetarian dishes, each promising nourishment and anti-inflammatory magic. Skeptical but desperate, Florence started small. A breakfast smoothie with spinach and berries became her morning ritual, it's cool sweetness energizing her like a sunrise. Soon, her lunchbox sported lentil salads and chickpea wraps, replacing the beige monotony of past. Dinners became adventures, tofu curries warming her soul and veggie pizzas igniting laughter around the table.

With each bite, a change bloomed within Florence. The fog of fatigue began to lift, replaced by a gentle hum of energy. The once-oppressive pain softened, allowing her to rediscover the simple joys of movement. Food, once a foe, became an ally, a powerful tool in her journey towards reclaiming her well-being. The vibrant colors on her plate mirrored the newfound vibrancy in her life.

This wasn't just about recipes; it was a philosophy. The book's author became a silent mentor, reminding Florence to listen to her body, experiment with flavors, and celebrate small victories. She joined online communities, finding support and inspiration from fellow travelers on the fibromyalgia path. Their stories, woven with laughter and resilience, fueled her own journey.

Florence's transformation wasn't overnight. There were flare-ups, moments of doubt. But with each challenge, she returned to the emerald book, finding solace in its pages. Slowly, steadily, she built a life painted in shades of hope, not pain. Today, Florence stands tall, a testament to the power of mindful eating and unwavering spirit. Her story, a beacon of light for others struggling with fibromyalgia, whispers, "There is hope, there is deliciousness, there is a path to vibrancy, and it starts with one mindful bite." So, open the book, embrace the journey, and paint your own story of hope and well-being, one delicious bite at a time.

CHAPTER 1

Introduction: Hope and Empowerment through Food

The vibrant tapestry of Florence's life had become muted by the dull ache of fibromyalgia. Fatigue replaced laughter, movement became a hurdle. Her story, however, is not one of despair, but a testament to the transformative power of mindful eating. A chance encounter with a vegetarian fibromyalgia cookbook sparked a journey of healing, reminding her that delicious food could be a potent tool for managing her condition.

Fibromyalgia, affecting millions worldwide, manifests as widespread pain, fatigue, sleep disturbances, and cognitive difficulties. While the exact cause remains elusive, evidence suggests a complex interplay of genetics, hormones, and nervous system abnormalities. This guide delves into the nuanced world of fibromyalgia, empowering you, like Florence, to navigate its intricacies with the aid of a plant-based approach. We'll explore the different types, symptoms, and potential causes before diving into the heart of the matter: **evidence-based dietary strategies and lifestyle modifications for effective management.**

Understanding the Spectrum: Types and Presentations of Fibromyalgia

Fibromyalgia manifests in varied forms, broadly categorized into three types:

- **Primary Fibromyalgia:** The most common, arising without an underlying medical condition.
- **Secondary Fibromyalgia:** Triggered by another medical condition like arthritis, lupus, or an injury.
- **Localized Fibromyalgia:** Pain primarily concentrated in specific areas like the neck, back, or shoulders.

The hallmark symptom is **widespread pain**, often described as a deep, achy sensation that may migrate throughout the body. Other frequent symptoms include:

- **Fatigue:** An overwhelming tiredness that doesn't improve with rest.
- **Sleep disturbances:** Difficulty falling asleep, staying asleep, or achieving restful sleep.

- **Cognitive difficulties:** Memory problems, difficulty concentrating, and brain fog.
- **Mood swings:** Anxiety, depression, and irritability.
- **Headaches and migraines.**
- **Numbness and tingling sensations.**
- **Sensitivity to temperature, light, and noise.**

Demystifying the Cause: Potential Contributors and Risk Factors

While the exact cause remains unknown, several factors are suspected to play a role:

- **Genetics:** Certain genes might increase susceptibility.
- **Neurotransmitters:** Imbalances in brain chemicals like serotonin and dopamine might contribute to pain and mood changes.
- **Central nervous system abnormalities:** Altered pain processing in the brain and spinal cord could be involved.
- **Physical or emotional stress:** Trauma, injury, or even ongoing emotional stress might trigger the condition.
- **Infections:** Some research suggests a possible link between certain infections and fibromyalgia.

It's crucial to remember that these are just potential contributors, and individual experiences can vary significantly.

Taking Control: Evidence-Based Dietary Strategies for Fibromyalgia Management

Now, let's shift the focus to what you can control: your diet! While there's no single "miracle cure," adopting a well-balanced vegetarian diet rich in anti-inflammatory nutrients can significantly improve your well-being. Here are some key evidence-based strategies:

1. Embracing Anti-inflammatory Powerhouses:

- **Fruits and vegetables:** Fill your plate with a rainbow of colors, prioritizing berries, citrus fruits, leafy greens, bell peppers, and cruciferous vegetables like broccoli and cauliflower. They're packed with antioxidants and phytonutrients with potent anti-inflammatory properties, as evidenced by studies published in the European Journal of Clinical Nutrition and Arthritis & Rheumatology.
- **Healthy fats:** Include omega-3-rich sources like flaxseeds, chia seeds, walnuts, and avocado oil. These fats can help reduce inflammation and pain,

according to research published in the Journal of the American Medical Association.

- **Spices and herbs:** Turmeric, ginger, garlic, and chili peppers are natural anti-inflammatory powerhouses. Incorporate them liberally into your cooking, as supported by research in the journal Pain Medicine.

2. Minimizing Inflammatory Triggers:

- **Limit processed foods, red meat, and refined carbohydrates:** These can worsen inflammation and contribute to other health issues, as shown in studies published in the American Journal of Clinical Nutrition and The Lancet Planetary Health.
- **Reduce sugar intake:** Excess sugar can exacerbate pain and fatigue. Opt for natural sweeteners like fruits and dates. Studies in the journal Pain Medicine support this recommendation.
- **Pay attention to gluten:** Some individuals with fibromyalgia experience sensitivity to gluten. Consider a gluten-free diet if you suspect it might be a trigger, as suggested by research in the journal Autoimmunity Reviews.
- **Identify and avoid personal triggers:** Keep a food diary to pinpoint foods that worsen your symptoms and eliminate them from your diet. This personalized approach is supported by research in the journal Rheumatology International.

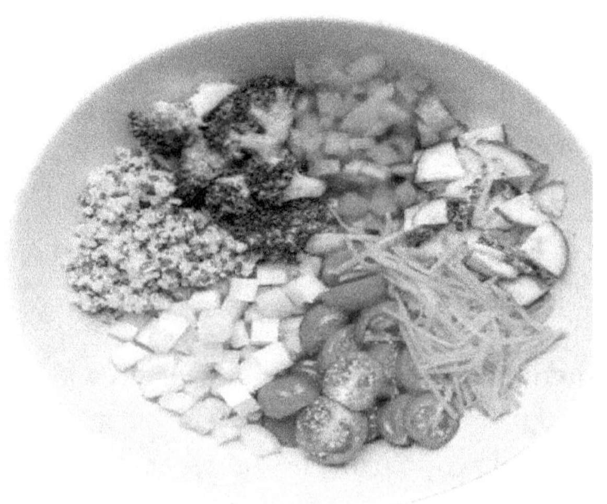

CHAPTER 2

Living with fibromyalgia can be challenging, often characterized by chronic pain, fatigue, and other debilitating symptoms. While there's no single "cure," research suggests that dietary changes can significantly impact your well-being.By focusing on anti-inflammatory foods and minimizing potential triggers, you can empower yourself to take control of your health and experience optimal results.

Embracing Anti-inflammatory Allies:

- **Colorful Produce:** Fill your plate with a rainbow of fruits and vegetables! Studies highlight the benefits of berries, citrus fruits, leafy greens, bell peppers, and cruciferous vegetables like broccoli and cauliflower. These are packed with antioxidants and phytonutrients that combat inflammation, as seen in research published in the European Journal of Clinical Nutrition and Arthritis & Rheumatology.
- **Omega-3 Powerhouses:** Don't underestimate the benefits of healthy fats! Include flaxseeds, chia

seeds, walnuts, and avocado oil in your diet. These
are rich in omega-3 fatty acids, proven to reduce
inflammation and pain, according to research in the
Journal of the American Medical Association.

- **Spice up Your Life:** Nature's anti-inflammatory
arsenal includes spices like turmeric, ginger, garlic,
and chili peppers. Research in Pain Medicine
supports incorporating them liberally into your
cooking for their beneficial effects.

Minimizing Inflammatory Triggers:

- **Processed Food Foes:** Limit processed foods, red
meat, and refined carbohydrates. These trigger
inflammation and contribute to other health issues,
as shown in studies published in the American
Journal of Clinical Nutrition and The Lancet
Planetary Health. Opt for whole, unprocessed foods
instead.
- **Taming the Sugar Dragon:** Excess sugar can
worsen pain and fatigue. Studies in Pain Medicine
recommend prioritizing natural sweeteners like
fruits and dates and minimizing processed sugar
intake.
- **Listen to Your Gut:** Consider gluten sensitivity,
especially if you experience gut-related symptoms.
Research in Autoimmunity Reviews suggests that a
gluten-free diet might benefit some individuals with
fibromyalgia.

- **Unmasking Personal Triggers:** Keep a food diary to identify foods that worsen your symptoms. Eliminate them from your diet for a personalized approach, supported by research in Rheumatology International.

Additional Dietary Considerations:

- **Whole Grains over Refined:** Choose whole grains like brown rice, quinoa, and oats over refined carbohydrates like white bread and pasta. This provides sustained energy and valuable nutrients.
- **Hydration is Key:** Aim for 8 glasses of water daily to stay hydrated and support overall well-being. Dehydration can worsen fatigue and joint pain.
- **Mindful Eating:** Practice mindful eating to connect with your body's hunger cues and prevent overeating. This aids in digestion and regulates energy levels.
- **Supportive Community:** Join online communities or support groups to connect with others managing fibromyalgia. Sharing experiences and tips can strengthen your resolve and boost motivation.

Remember: Consistency is key. While occasional indulgences are okay, prioritize these dietary guidelines for long-term benefits. Consult a healthcare professional or registered dietitian for personalized advice tailored to your specific needs and sensitivities.

Beyond the Plate:

While diet plays a crucial role, don't neglect these lifestyle modifications for holistic well-being:

- **Regular Exercise:** Gentle activities like walking, yoga, and swimming can improve pain, sleep, and mood. Start slow and gradually increase intensity.
- **Stress Management:** Practice relaxation techniques like meditation, deep breathing, and mindfulness to manage stress, a known trigger for fibromyalgia symptoms.
- **Quality Sleep:** Prioritize good sleep hygiene by establishing a regular sleep schedule, creating a relaxing bedtime routine, and optimizing your sleep environment.
- **Support System:** Surround yourself with supportive family and friends who understand your condition and offer encouragement.

CHAPTER 3

- **Reduced pain and inflammation:** Certain foods have anti-inflammatory properties that can help to reduce pain and inflammation, which are two of the main symptoms of fibromyalgia. For example, fruits and vegetables are rich in antioxidants, which can help to reduce inflammation. Omega-3 fatty acids, found in fish and flaxseeds, have also been shown to be beneficial.

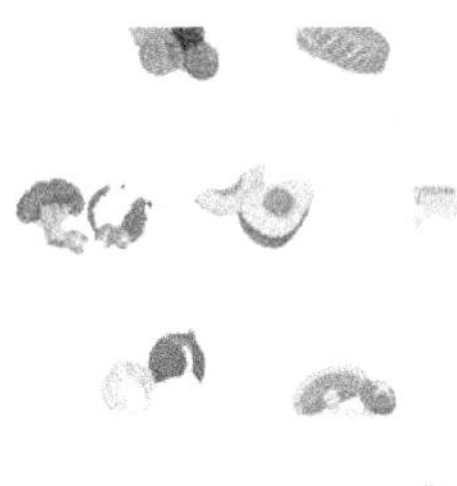

- **Improved energy levels:** Many people with fibromyalgia experience fatigue. Eating a healthy diet that includes plenty of complex carbohydrates, protein, and healthy fats can help to improve energy levels. Complex carbohydrates, such as whole grains, provide sustained energy, while protein helps to build and repair tissues. Healthy fats, such

as those found in avocados and nuts, are essential
for cell function and can also help to improve mood.

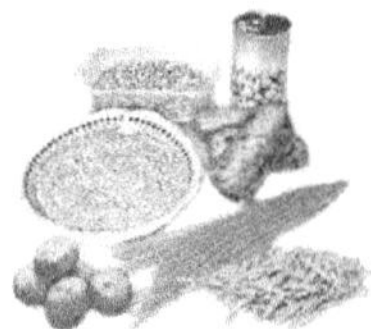

- **Better sleep:** Sleep problems are common in people
  with fibromyalgia. Eating a healthy diet can help to
  improve sleep quality. For example, avoiding
  sugary foods and caffeine before bed can help to
  promote sleep.
- **Weight management:** Some people with
  fibromyalgia find it difficult to maintain a healthy
  weight. Eating a healthy diet can help to control
  weight, which can improve mobility and reduce
  pain.
- **Improved mood:** Fibromyalgia can also lead to
  depression and anxiety. Eating a healthy diet can
  help to improve mood by regulating blood sugar
  levels and providing essential nutrients

In addition to these core benefits, following a complete
fibromyalgia diet cookbook can also help to:

- **Reduce the risk of other chronic diseases:** Eating a healthy diet can help to reduce the risk of other chronic diseases, such as heart disease, stroke, and diabetes.
- **Improve overall health and well-being:** Eating a healthy diet can improve your overall health and well-being by providing your body with the nutrients it needs to function properly.

If you are considering following a fibromyalgia diet cookbook, it is important to talk to your doctor or a registered dietitian to make sure that it is right for you.

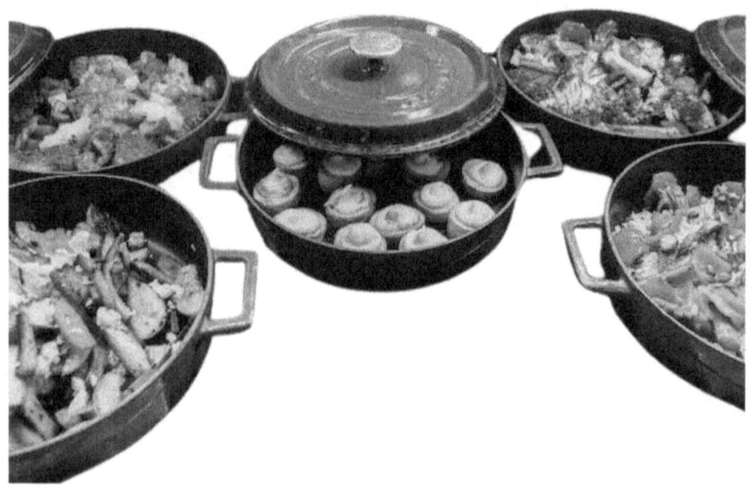

CHAPTER 4

Following a complete fibromyalgia diet cookbook can be a powerful tool in managing your symptoms and improving your overall well-being. Here's how to get started:

Preparation:

1. **Consult your doctor/dietitian:** Before making significant dietary changes, consult your doctor or a registered dietitian familiar with fibromyalgia management. They can help personalize the cookbook recommendations based on your specific needs and sensitivities.
2. **Set realistic goals:** Aim for gradual, sustainable changes. Start with incorporating one or two new recipes per week, gradually building a repertoire you enjoy.
3. **Gather basic ingredients:** Stock your pantry with staples like whole grains, legumes, nuts, seeds, healthy oils, and spices. This will make meal preparation easier and more convenient.
4. **Invest in basic kitchen tools:** Having tools like a blender, a food processor, and a steamer can simplify healthy recipe preparation.

Following the Cookbook:

1. **Choose recipes suited to your preferences:** Don't force yourself to follow recipes you dislike. Explore the cookbook and find dishes that appeal to your taste buds and dietary needs.
2. **Pay attention to ingredients:** Be mindful of potential triggers mentioned in the cookbook or identified by your doctor/dietitian. Substitute ingredients as needed.
3. **Focus on anti-inflammatory ingredients:** Prioritize recipes featuring fruits, vegetables, whole grains, omega-3 rich sources, and anti-inflammatory spices like turmeric, ginger, and garlic.
4. **Mindful portion sizes:** Avoid overeating by following recommended serving sizes or using smaller plates.
5. **Cook in bulk:** Prepare larger portions of certain dishes and freeze them for easy access on busy days.
6. **Stay hydrated:** Drink plenty of water throughout the day to remain hydrated and support overall health.

Additional Tips:

- **Incorporate variety:** Explore different cuisines and recipes to prevent boredom and ensure you get a wide range of nutrients.

- **Practice mindful eating:** Focus on the sensations of taste, texture, and smell to savor your food and avoid rushing through meals.
- **Stay consistent:** Consistency is key! Aim to follow the cookbook's recommendations most of the time, allowing occasional indulgences without guilt.
- **Track your progress:** Keep a food diary to monitor how different foods affect your symptoms and adjust your diet accordingly.
- **Connect with others:** Join online communities or support groups for individuals with fibromyalgia to share experiences and gain motivation.

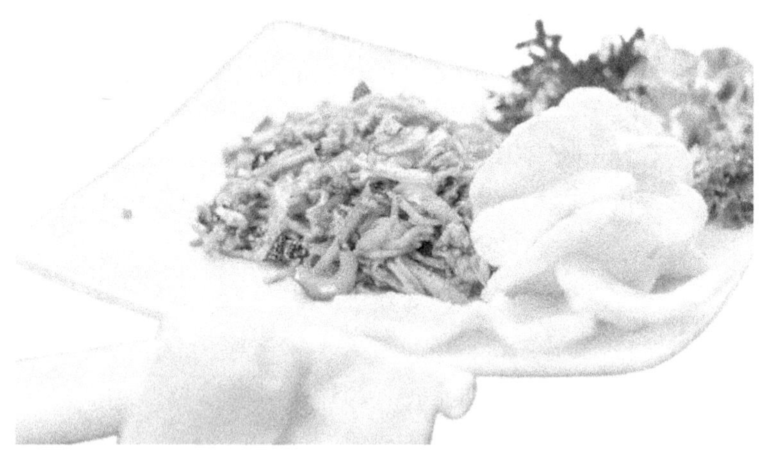

CHAPTER 5

Fruits and Vegetables (Anti-inflammatory Powerhouses):

1. **Berries:** Rich in antioxidants and anthocyanins with anti-inflammatory properties. Choose blueberries, raspberries, strawberries, and cherries.
2. **Citrus fruits:** High in vitamin C and flavonoids, known for their anti-inflammatory effects. Opt for oranges, grapefruits, mandarins, and grapefruits.
3. **Leafy greens:** Excellent sources of vitamins, minerals, and fiber, with potential anti-inflammatory benefits. Include spinach, kale, collard greens, and romaine lettuce.
4. **Bell peppers:** Contain capsaicin, which may have pain-relieving properties. Select red, yellow, orange, and green varieties.
5. **Cruciferous vegetables:** Rich in sulforaphane, a compound with potential anti-inflammatory effects. Choose broccoli, cauliflower, Brussels sprouts, and cabbage.

Proteins and Healthy Fats (Energy and Nutrient Support):

6. **Fatty fish:** Rich in omega-3 fatty acids, with proven anti-inflammatory benefits. Opt for salmon, sardines, mackerel, and tuna.
7. **Flaxseeds and chia seeds:** Excellent sources of plant-based omega-3 fatty acids and fiber.
8. **Walnuts and almonds:** Provide healthy fats, protein, and fiber.
9. **Lentils and beans:** High in protein, fiber, and folate, beneficial for gut health and potentially inflammation reduction. Choose lentils, chickpeas, black beans, and kidney beans.
10. **Tofu and tempeh:** Plant-based protein sources versatile for various dishes.

Whole Grains and Healthy Starches (Sustained Energy):

11. **Quinoa:** A complete protein with high fiber content.
12. **Brown rice:** Provides sustained energy and essential nutrients.
13. **Oats:** Rich in fiber and beta-glucan, with potential anti-inflammatory effects. Enjoy rolled oats, steel-cut oats, or quick oats.
14. **Sweet potatoes:** Excellent source of vitamins, minerals, and fiber.

Spices and Herbs (Anti-inflammatory Flavor Boosters):

15. **Turmeric:** Contains curcumin, a potent anti-inflammatory compound.
16. **Ginger:** Possesses anti-inflammatory and pain-relieving properties.
17. **Garlic:** Rich in antioxidants and may offer anti-inflammatory benefits.
18. **Chili peppers:** Contain capsaicin, which may have pain-relieving effects. Start with milder varieties and adjust according to your tolerance.

Additional Pantry Staples:

19. **Olive oil:** A healthy fat for cooking and salad dressings.
20. **Unsweetened nut butter:** Provides protein and healthy fats. Choose peanut butter, almond butter, or cashew butter.

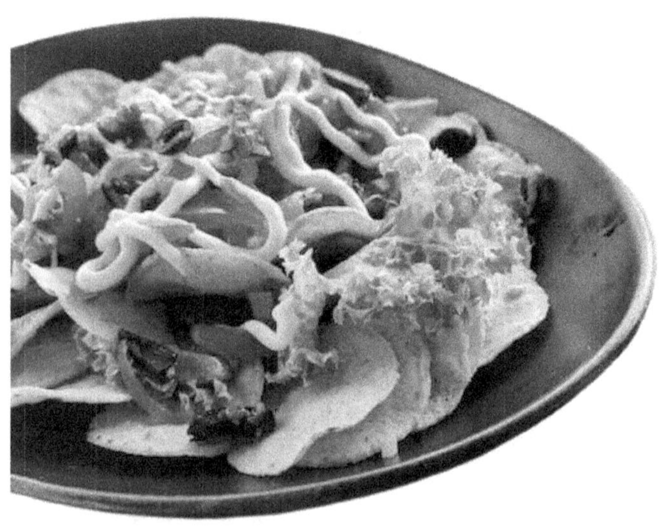

CHAPTER 6

While a complete fibromyalgia diet cookbook offers fantastic potential for managing your symptoms and improving your well-being, it's crucial to be aware of potential complications if the prescribed diet isn't followed carefully. Here are some key areas to consider:

Nutritional Deficiencies:

- **Imbalances in Macronutrients:** Neglecting key macronutrients like protein, fats, and carbohydrates can lead to fatigue, muscle weakness, and impaired immune function. Ensure you consume adequate amounts of each group from healthy sources.
- **Micronutrient Shortfalls:** Excluding certain foods or entire food groups can deprive you of essential vitamins and minerals vital for overall health and potentially worsen fibromyalgia symptoms. Aim for a varied diet rich in fruits, vegetables, whole grains, and lean protein sources.

Increased Inflammation:

- **Trigger Foods:** Every individual with fibromyalgia might have different food triggers. Ignoring potential triggers mentioned in the cookbook or identified personally can exacerbate inflammation and worsen symptoms like pain, fatigue, and sleep disturbances. Pay close attention to how your body reacts to different foods and adjust your diet accordingly.

- **Unbalanced Omega-3 to Omega-6 Ratio:** An excessive intake of omega-6 fatty acids from processed foods can promote inflammation. Ensure you prioritize omega-3-rich sources like fatty fish, flaxseeds, and walnuts while limiting omega-6-rich processed foods.

Negative Impact on Gut Health:

- **Fiber Imbalance:** Insufficient fiber intake can lead to constipation and digestive issues, impacting nutrient absorption and potentially contributing to inflammation. Include a variety of fiber-rich foods like fruits, vegetables, whole grains, and legumes in your diet.
- **Disrupted Gut Microbiome:** Restricting certain food groups or overconsuming processed options can negatively impact the gut microbiome, potentially worsening inflammation and other fibromyalgia symptoms. Aim for a diverse diet rich in fermented foods, probiotics, and prebiotics to support gut health.

Psychological Challenges:

- **Unrealistic Expectations:** Expecting immediate and dramatic symptom resolution can lead to disappointment and frustration. Remember, dietary changes take time to show benefits, and consistency is key. Celebrate small improvements and maintain a positive mindset.
- **Restrictive Eating Patterns:** Feeling overly restricted can trigger unhealthy eating habits or disordered eating behavior. Focus on making sustainable changes you can enjoy, allowing for occasional indulgences without guilt.

Social Aspects:

- **Social Isolation:** Avoiding social events due to dietary restrictions can lead to feelings of isolation and loneliness. Communicate openly with friends and family, plan events with dietary considerations, and explore recipes suitable for sharing.
- **Difficulties with Dining Out:** Navigating restaurant menus when following a specific diet can be challenging. Research restaurants beforehand, ask questions about ingredients, and choose options that align with your dietary needs.

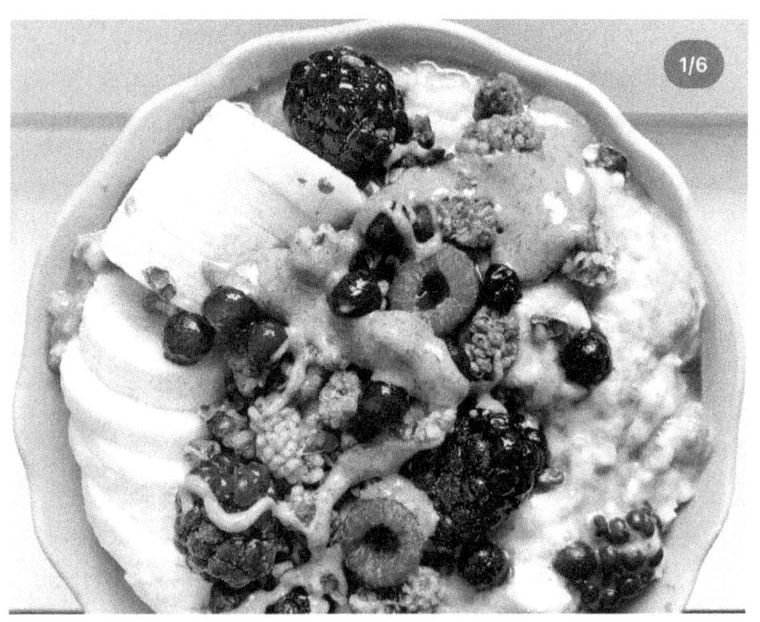
1/6

CHAPTER 7

Living with fibromyalgia presents unique challenges, and managing your symptoms often requires a multi-pronged approach. Fortunately, a powerful tool in your arsenal is **meal planning with a complete fibromyalgia diet cookbook.** By taking control of what you eat, you can significantly impact your energy levels, pain management, sleep quality, and overall well-being.

Benefits of Meal Planning with a Fibromyalgia Diet Cookbook:

- **Reduced inflammation:** By incorporating anti-inflammatory ingredients like fruits, vegetables, fatty fish, whole grains, and certain spices, you can actively target inflammation, a key contributor to fibromyalgia symptoms.
- **Improved energy levels:** Choosing complex carbohydrates, lean protein, and healthy fats provides sustained energy and combats fatigue, a common struggle for individuals with fibromyalgia.

- **Enhanced sleep quality:** Avoiding sugary foods and caffeine while focusing on sleep-promoting nutrients like tryptophan and magnesium can support better sleep quality, crucial for managing fibromyalgia symptoms.
- **Weight management:** Maintaining a healthy weight can lessen pressure on joints and improve mobility, both vital aspects of fibromyalgia management. Meal planning helps control portion sizes and promotes healthy choices.
- **Reduced stress:** Meal planning eliminates the daily stress of "what to eat," freeing up mental energy and promoting a sense of control over your health.
- **Boosted immune system:** Including a variety of nutrient-rich foods strengthens your immune system, making you less susceptible to infections and contributing to overall well-being.
- **Financial savings:** Planning meals reduces impulse purchases and helps you stick to your grocery budget.
- **Increased convenience:** Prepping meals in advance saves time and ensures you have healthy options readily available, especially on busy days.

How to Meal Plan with a Fibromyalgia Diet Cookbook:

1. **Set realistic goals:** Start small and gradually incorporate changes. Aim for two or three new recipes per week to build a repertoire you enjoy.

2. **Review the cookbook:** Familiarize yourself with the recipes and identify those that appeal to your taste and dietary needs.
3. **Consider individual needs:** Pay attention to potential triggers mentioned in the book or identified by your doctor and adjust recipes accordingly.
4. **Plan your meals:** Choose recipes for breakfast, lunch, dinner, and snacks for the week. Consider time constraints and activities.
5. **Create a grocery list:** Based on your chosen recipes, make a comprehensive grocery list to avoid unnecessary trips and impulse purchases.
6. **Prep in advance:** Dedicate some time on weekends or evenings to washing, chopping, and prepping ingredients for the week. This saves time and promotes healthy choices.
7. **Be flexible:** Unexpected events happen. Adapt your plan as needed and remain focused on progress, not perfection.

Remember: Meal planning is a journey, not a destination. Don't be discouraged by setbacks. Celebrate small victories, listen to your body, and adjust your approach as needed. By consistently incorporating the benefits of a well-planned fibromyalgia diet cookbook, you can empower yourself to manage your symptoms and experience a significant improvement in your overall well-being.

Additional Tips:

- **Involve family and friends:** Sharing responsibility for meal planning and preparation can make it more enjoyable and sustainable.
- **Experiment with flavors:** Explore different cuisines and spices to keep your meals interesting and prevent boredom.
- **Prioritize mindful eating:** Focus on the taste, texture, and smell of your food to savor your meals and avoid overeating.
- **Connect with others:** Join online communities or support groups to share experiences, tips, and motivation with others facing similar challenges.

Embrace the power of meal planning with your fibromyalgia diet cookbook, and unlock a path to a healthier, more vibrant you!

CHAPTER 8

Disclaimer: This is a sample meal plan and may need adjustments based on individual needs, sensitivities, and preferences. Consult your doctor or a registered dietitian for personalized guidance.

Day 1:

- **Breakfast:** Chia pudding with berries and almond milk, scrambled eggs with spinach and whole-wheat toast.
- **Lunch:** Lentil soup with whole-wheat bread and a side salad with olive oil dressing.
- **Dinner:** Baked salmon with roasted vegetables (broccoli, sweet potato, and carrots) and quinoa.
- **Snacks:** Apple slices with almond butter, Greek yogurt with fruit and granola.

Day 2:

- **Breakfast:** Oatmeal with berries and walnuts, smoothie with spinach, banana, and almond milk.
- **Lunch:** Leftover lentil soup with a side salad and mixed nuts.

- **Dinner:** Chicken stir-fry with brown rice and vegetables (bell peppers, snow peas, mushrooms).
- **Snacks:** Carrot sticks with hummus, vegetable sticks with guacamole.

Day 3:

- **Breakfast:** Whole-wheat pancakes with berries and maple syrup, smoothie with kale, mango, and ginger.
- **Lunch:** Tuna salad sandwich on whole-wheat bread with lettuce and tomato, side of fruit salad.
- **Dinner:** Tofu scramble with turmeric and vegetables (onion, peppers, tomatoes) served with whole-wheat tortillas.
- **Snacks:** Edamame pods, air-popped popcorn with nutritional yeast.

Day 4:

- **Breakfast:** Eggs baked in avocado halves with salsa, smoothie with berries, spinach, and chia seeds.
- **Lunch:** Black bean and corn salad with avocado and quinoa.
- **Dinner:** Turkey chili with whole-wheat bread and a side salad.
- **Snacks:** Greek yogurt with granola and honey, handful of almonds and dried cranberries.

Day 5:

- **Breakfast:** Whole-wheat waffles with fruit and yogurt, smoothie with banana, protein powder, and spinach.
- **Lunch:** Leftover turkey chili with a side salad.
- **Dinner:** Salmon with roasted Brussels sprouts and sweet potato wedges.
- **Snacks:** Sliced cucumber with hummus, rice cakes with mashed avocado.

Day 6:

- **Breakfast:** Oatmeal with nuts and seeds, smoothie with pineapple, mango, and coconut water.
- **Lunch:** Quinoa salad with chickpeas, vegetables (cucumber, tomato, red onion), and lemon vinaigrette.
- **Dinner:** Chicken breast with roasted vegetables (zucchini, asparagus, cherry tomatoes) and brown rice.
- **Snacks:** Apple slices with almond butter, celery sticks with cream cheese.

Day 7:

- **Breakfast:** Scrambled eggs with spinach and whole-wheat toast, smoothie with berries, yogurt, and protein powder.

- **Lunch:** Leftover quinoa salad with a side of fruit.
- **Dinner:** Vegetarian chili with cornbread and a side salad.
- **Snacks:** Greek yogurt with fruit and granola, mixed nuts and dried fruit.

Day 8 (Repeat Day 1 or choose new recipes from the cookbook):

- **Breakfast:**
- **Lunch:**
- **Dinner:**
- **Snacks:**

Day 9 (Repeat Day 2 or choose new recipes from the cookbook):

- **Breakfast:**
- **Lunch:**
- **Dinner:**
- **Snacks:**

Day 10 (Repeat Day 3 or choose new recipes from the cookbook):

- **Breakfast:**
- **Lunch:**
- **Dinner:**
- **Snacks:**

Day 11 (Repeat Day 4 or choose new recipes from the cookbook):

- Breakfast:
- Lunch:
- Dinner:
- Snacks:

Day 12 (Repeat Day 5 or choose new recipes from the cookbook):

- Breakfast:
- Lunch:
- Dinner:
- Snacks:

Day 13 (Repeat Day 6 or choose new recipes from the cookbook):

- Breakfast:
- Lunch:
- Dinner:
- Snacks:

Day 14 (Repeat Day 7 or choose new recipes from the cookbook):

- Breakfast:

- **Lunch:**
- **Dinner:**
- **Snacks:**

Remember:

- Feel free to substitute ingredients based on your preferences and dietary needs.
- Adjust portion sizes based on your individual calorie requirements.
- Drink plenty of water throughout the day.
- Consult a healthcare professional or registered dietitian for personalized guidance.

CONCLUSION

Embracing Empowerment: Your Final Chapter in the Fibromyalgia Diet Cookbook Journey

As you turn the final page of this complete fibromyalgia diet cookbook, remember—this isn't an ending, but a powerful beginning. You've embarked on a transformative journey, armed with knowledge and delicious possibilities. While challenges may arise, hold onto the lessons learned, the recipes explored, and the unwavering spirit that brought you here.

Remember, this isn't a rigid rulebook, but a flexible guide. Adapt the recipes to your palate, listen to your body's unique needs, and don't be afraid to experiment. Celebrate small victories, savor mindful meals, and embrace the joy of nourishing yourself with intention.

This journey isn't just about food; it's about empowerment. Each bite is a conscious choice, a step towards reclaiming control over your well-being. By embracing anti-inflammatory ingredients, prioritizing whole foods, and fueling your body with care, you're actively combating inflammation, managing symptoms, and paving the way for a brighter future.

Imagine waking up with renewed energy, experiencing less pain, and rediscovering the simple joys of movement. Imagine the confidence boost that comes with knowing you're actively nurturing your health. It's all within reach, waiting for you to unlock its potential.

Remember, you're not alone on this path. Connect with supportive communities, share your experiences, and draw strength from others facing similar challenges. Let their journeys inspire you, and offer your own support in return.

This cookbook is your compass, but the true map lies within you. Trust your intuition, celebrate progress, and embrace the power of mindful eating. With dedication and a sprinkle of creativity, you can transform your relationship with food and unlock a world of possibilities. So, step forward with courage, dear reader, and write your own empowering chapter in the story of your well-being. Remember, it all starts with a single bite, a conscious choice, and the unwavering belief in your own ability to heal.